MANAGING CORONARY HEART DISEASE

Detail on Causes, Management, Treatment and More

BY

WM J. FRAZIER

COPYRIGHT©2020

COPYRIGHT

No part of this, publication may be reproduced, distributed, or transmitted in any form or by any means, including photocopy, recording or other electronic or mechanical methods or by any information storage and retrieval system without the prior written permission of the publisher, except in a case of very brief quotations embodied in critical reviews and certain other noncommercial uses permitted by copyright law.

TABLE OF CONTENT

CHAPTER 1

A LITTLE ABOUT CHD

CHAPTER 2

MORE ABOUT CORONARY HEART DISEASE

CHAPTER 3

POSSIBLE CAUSES OF CORONARY HEART DISEASE (CHD)

CHAPTER 4

POSSIBLE TREATMENTS OF CORONARY DISEASE

CHAPTER 6

RISKS FACTORS AND MANAGEMENT OF CORONARY DISEASE

THE END

CHAPTER 1

A LITTLE ABOUT CHD

One of the very troubling situations plaguing people of different parts of the world is the

Coronary Heart Disease (CHD). It's so serious that if not properly and quickly diagnosed and managed the patient dies.

As you probably know already, the heart is a muscle about the size of a human fist. Blood flows from the heart, moves to the lungs to accumulate oxygen. The blood now with oxygen is transported to other organs and parts of the body through the arteries.

The Coronary Heart Diseases (CHD) is a condition that occurs in people when cholesterol builds up on the wall of the artery, causing blockage. The arteries become constricted hindering blood flow to the heart muscle.

Coronary Heart Disease (CHD) is capable of resulting to shortness of breath, and if as a result of this there isn't enough oxygen for the heart and other organs may lead to other severe health conditions and the patient may start dying.

CHAPTER 2

MORE ABOUT CORONARY HEART DISEASE

There're some things about this disease that one must not forget at anytime.

The Coronary Heart Diseases (CHD) is a condition that occurs in people when cholesterol builds up on the wall of the artery, causing blockage. The arteries become constricted hindering blood flow to the heart muscle.

Coronary Heart Disease (CHD) is capable of resulting to shortness of breath, and if as a result of this there isn't enough oxygen for the heart and other organs may lead to other severe health conditions and the patient may start dying.

This disease in most cases lead to ANGINA or MYOCARDIAL INFARCTION.

- Angina: happens when the thinness of the coronary artery, results in severe chest pain or rigidity in the chest. This therefore makes walking, climbing stairs, lifting heavy objects and other exercises difficult. In most cases this condition is temporary.

- Myocardial Infarction: this is a situation that happens due to total blockage of the coronary artery by blood clot (Thrombosis). Because of this, the heart muscle after the blockage dies. This is the for the most part of the world common type of heart disease, as it is the cause of over 370,000 deaths every year in the United States which accounts for.

As you probably know already, the heart is a muscle about the size of a human fist. Blood flows from the heart, moves to the lungs to accumulate oxygen. The blood now with oxygen is transported to other organs and parts of the body through the arteries. The process of movement of blood is known as circulation.

The coronary arteries are the heart's mode of transporting or moving blood vessels. It's this coronary arteries that also distributes oxygen to the heart muscles. Once it happens that the coronary arteries slims down, it diminishes the delivery of oxygen-rich blood to the heart especially when carrying out physical actions of the body.

At the early stage of this drop in oxygen-rich blood flow, there might be no signs or symptoms; but as fat and other stuffs pile up, you start getting signs and symptoms.

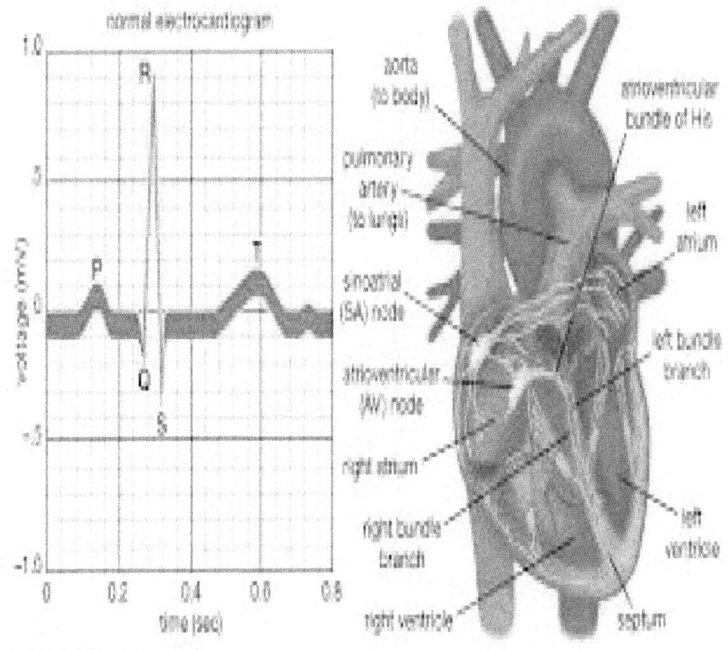

CHAPTER 3

POSSIBLE CAUSES OF CORONARY HEART DISEASE (CHD)

Wound or harm to the interior layer of a coronary artery is the start of a coronary heart disease. The harm in the interior layer of the coronary artery makes fatty dumps to pile up where the wound is. These dumps are made up of cholesterol and other wastes. This buildup of dumps is referred to as atherosclerosis.

When there're wounds, platelets will cluster at that place trying to fix the tampered blood vessel. This cluster unintentionally blocks the artery, reducing or blocking blood flow and leading to a heart attack.

Symptoms of Coronary Heart Disease

ANGINA: The chief signs and symptoms of angina is pain in the chest, neck, jaw, arms, shoulders, throat, back or teeth. One usually feels this pain when doing heavy works and stops once you rest. Most times you first feel it behind the breastbone. One may at times notice numbness or heaviness in the arms, the symptoms increases after a meal or when in the cold or climbing a hill or into a strong wind (peripheral vasoconstriction higher oxygen demand).

Myocardial infarction (Heart Attack): The chief sign or symptom of myocardial infarction is pain in the chest or restlessness. This may look like same symptom with Angina but they are not, because it doesn't just go by resting or relaxing and lasts for hours. It's mostly caused by the death of the heart muscle because of lack of blood and oxygen.

Other symptoms of Myocardial infarction (heart attack) include:

1. Uneasiness around the chest, light or severe chest pain
2. Cough
3. Dizziness
4. Difficulty breathing
5. Paleness in the face
6. Constant feeling of unwell.
7. sickness and vomiting
8. Restlessness
9. Sweaty and sticky skin

This situation is capable of leading to death as it causes lifelong damage to the heart muscle.

CHAPTER 4

POSSIBLE TREATMENTS OF CORONARY DISEASE

The Coronary heart disease is known not to have a treatment today; however it can be excellently managed for better health.

Some of the known management strategies like Adjustment of dangerous lifestyles e.g stop smoking cigarette, try eating healthier meals and regular exercises.

There are also some known medical procedures that are known to be effective. These include:

- Statins: except the patient has high cholesterol issue, this medication is most effective for coronary heart disease.

- Aspirin: taking aspirin reduces the activity of blood clothing which causes angina.

- Beta blockers: this reduces blood pressure and heart beats, mostly among heart attack victims.

- Nitroglycerin patches, sprays or tablets: these substances manage chest pain by expanding the coronary arteries and sending enough blood to the heart.

- Angiotensin-converting enzyme (ACE) inhibitors: The above does the job of lessening blood pressure and slowing down or stopping the growth of CHD.

- Calcium channel blockers: This enlarges the coronary arteries, letting more blood flow to the heart, therefore reducing high blood pressure.

CHAPTER 6

RISKS FACTORS AND MANAGEMENT OF CORONARY DISEASE

Some of the known risk factors of coronary heart disease are:

- Hypertension

- Smoking
- Diabetes mellitus
- Obesity
- No physical exercise

Management of Coronary Disease

Angina: patients suffering from Angina can manage the condition by doing the following:

1. Take on and attend classes on health education about eradicating or reducing the risk factors associated with CHD.

2. Customary taking of medications like the triturate, beta blockers etc. for relieve or prevention of pain.

3. Surgery especially in extreme cases.

Heart Attack: Heart Attack on the other hand can be managed well if patients do the following:

1. Constant and update health education will help to reduce the effect of CHD.

2. It's important to have regular bed rest before and during hospitalization.

3. By receiving maximum medical attention from a specialist.

4. Steady healing.

Types of angina

- Stable angina: this is characterized by a discomfort that may last for a while, feeling like gas or indigestion. It occurs mostly if the heart works unusually harder. E.g during exercise and it reoccurs during a period of a month or years; but can be taken care of by regular resting or medication.

- Unstable angina: this condition is as a result of blood clots in the coronary artery. It happens at times when relaxing, lasts longer and may become worse over time.

- Variant angina: this class of angina happens when resting and is usually severe. It is a result of a spasm in an artery which makes it tighten and narrow, disturbing blood delivery to the heart. Exposure to cold, stress, medications, smoking or cocaine, are capable of starting or causing it.

THE END

www.ingramcontent.com/pod-product-compliance
Lightning Source LLC
Chambersburg PA
CBHW050329220526
45465CB00005B/2192